CHRISTOPHER F. CAMPBELL

How Sleep Recharges Your Body And Mind

The Holistic Guide on sleep with Essential Strategies for Reducing Stress, Increasing Energy and Living a Healthier Life

Contents

Introduction   v

Understanding Your Sleep   1

   Sleep cycles and stages   2

   Factors that affect your sleep patterns   3

   Indicators of sleep quality and quantity
issues   4

   Assessing your individual sleep needs   5

   Weekly Sleeping Tracker   7

Establishing a Bedtime Routine   10

   Ways to wind down before bed   11

   Creating a calm, restful sleep environment   12

   Developing a consistent sleep-wake sched-
ule   13

   Reducing screen time and exposure to blue light   14

Relaxing the Mind and Body for Better Sleep   16

   Stress management techniques   17

   Gentle yoga and stretching before bed   18

   Mindfulness and meditation practices   19

Nutrition and Lifestyle Strategies for Quality Sleep   21

   The role of diet in sleep   22

   Hydration and avoiding late-night drinks   23

   Exercise and activity levels   25

   Caffeine, nicotine and other substances   26

Common Sleep Disorders   29

Insomnia   30

Sleep apnea   31

Restless legs syndrome   32

Narcolepsy   33

Putting It All Together   35

Customizing a self-care routine for better sleep   36

Overcoming obstacles and maintaining changes   38

Achieving holistic wellness through quality sleep   40

Conclusion   43

Introduction

Wake up refreshed and ready to take on the day. How many of us can honestly say we feel this way? In our fast-paced world where "busy" has become a badge of honor, it's easy to overlook something as basic as sleep. But the truth is, getting adequate, quality sleep is crucial for our mental, physical and emotional well-being.

As a holistic health coach, I've seen firsthand the impact of poor sleep on my clients. Many struggle with low energy, mood issues, difficulty focusing and even weight gain—all consequences of not getting enough of this essential function. And it's more than just feeling tired—lack of sleep can seriously impact our health over the long run by increasing risks for diseases like diabetes, heart disease and obesity.

The goals of this guidebook are to educate you on why sleep matters so much, uncover any roadblocks to your quality slumber, and provide natural strategies to improve your sleep hygiene and establish a more restful routine. Inside you will find tools and techniques from Ayurveda, Chinese medicine, mindfulness practices and more to help you unwind your body and mind each night. With custom lifestyle tips and natural remedies, you'll discover an approach tailored just for you.

By prioritizing sleep as seriously as diet and exercise, you can reap holistic benefits like reduced stress, increased energy levels and an overall better quality of life. Use this handbook as your personal sleep coach to reset your circadian rhythm, support restorative rest, and wake feeling truly refreshed each morning. When we nourish our bodies and minds with quality sleep each night, we give ourselves the gift of health, wellness and peak performance throughout each new day.

What is sleep and why is it important

What exactly is sleep, and why is it so crucial for our well-being? Simply put, sleep is a natural, vital process that allows our minds and bodies to restore and recharge overnight.

Although it may seem like a passive activity, sleep is anything but resting. While we slumber, our brain waves and breathing slow down as our bodies repair cells, form new pathways in the brain, strengthen the immune system and produce important hormones. Without sufficient sleep, all these important restoration processes are disrupted.

There are two main types of sleep—non-REM and REM sleep. Non-REM sleep helps the body relax and prepares us for dreaming, while REM (rapid eye movement) sleep is when most vivid dreams occur as the brain consolidates memories and processes emotions. Getting adequate time in each sleep stage is integral for overall health.

Research shows sleep impacts virtually every system in our bodies. Not only does it boost our mood, learning and memory, but it also regulates appetite hormones, supports a healthy metabolism and cardiac function. Lack of quality slumber has even been tied to an increased risk of obesity, diabetes, depression and certain cancers over time.

Getting just 30 minutes less than our individual need on a consistent basis can cognitively impact us like being drunk! That's why prioritizing sufficient shut-eye is just as important as nourishment and physical fitness for holistic wellness. Our sleep directly fuels how we feel, think and function throughout each new day.

Common sleep issues facing modern society

Insomnia - Trouble falling or staying asleep affects approximately 30% of adults at some point. Stress, lifestyle habits, and certain medications can all contribute to insomnia.

Sleep Deprivation - Our 24/7 work culture means too many people don't get the recommended 7-9 hours per night. Chronic sleep loss has serious health consequences over time.

Shift Work Disorder - Late nights, early mornings, and changing schedules disrupt the body's circadian rhythm for those in jobs like healthcare, transportation, hospitality.

Technology Overuse - Devices emit blue light that suppresses melatonin production and makes it harder to fall asleep. Social media and screens right before bed are especially disruptive.

Medical Conditions - Obstructive sleep apnea, restless leg syndrome, chronic pain, asthma and acid reflux can all disturb quality slumber if conditions are uncontrolled.

Caffeine & Stimulant Dependence - Many people rely on coffee, tea, soda or energy drinks to power through busy days but caffeine intake too close to bedtime causes problems falling asleep and staying asleep.

Irregular Bedtimes - Without consistent wake up and sleeping times, our body's clock has trouble regulating the sleep-wake cycle according to light and darkness cues in the environment.

Lack of Routine - Many of us underestimate how winding down rituals, exercise, diet and managing stress impact sleep quality long-term with consistent routines.

The holistic benefits of adequate, quality sleep

Here are some of the holistic benefits our bodies and minds experience with adequate, quality sleep each night:

- Improved Mood - Deep sleep regulates serotonin and other neurotransmitters to promote relaxation and boost mood. Lack of sleep can contribute to depression and anxiety.

- Lean Metabolism - Growth hormone release during sleep supports fat burning and weight management by regulating appetite hormones like leptin and ghrelin.

- Reduced Stress Levels - Sleep allows the endocrine and nervous systems to unwind from stressors. Melatonin produced at night has antioxidant properties that counteract oxidative stress.

- Sharper Cognition - While we slumber, the brain consolidates memories and clears out toxins to boost focus, concentration, and overall brain performance when awake.

- Stronger Immunity - Deep sleep bolsters the immune system as white blood cell and antibody production increases overnight. Fatigue hinders our body's immunity.

- Better Heart Health - Studies show insufficient sleep raises blood pressure and risk for heart attack, stroke and cardiovascular disease over the long run.

- Healthy Aging - Deep sleep supports the production of new cells, protein folding and other reparative processes to slow age-related cognitive decline.

- Higher Energy Levels - Waking rested allows our organs, glands and systems to properly fuel our days with focus, motivation and productivity.

Adequate, quality sleep forms the foundation for holistic wellness by supporting our physical, mental-emotional and cellular health every single night.

Understanding Your Sleep

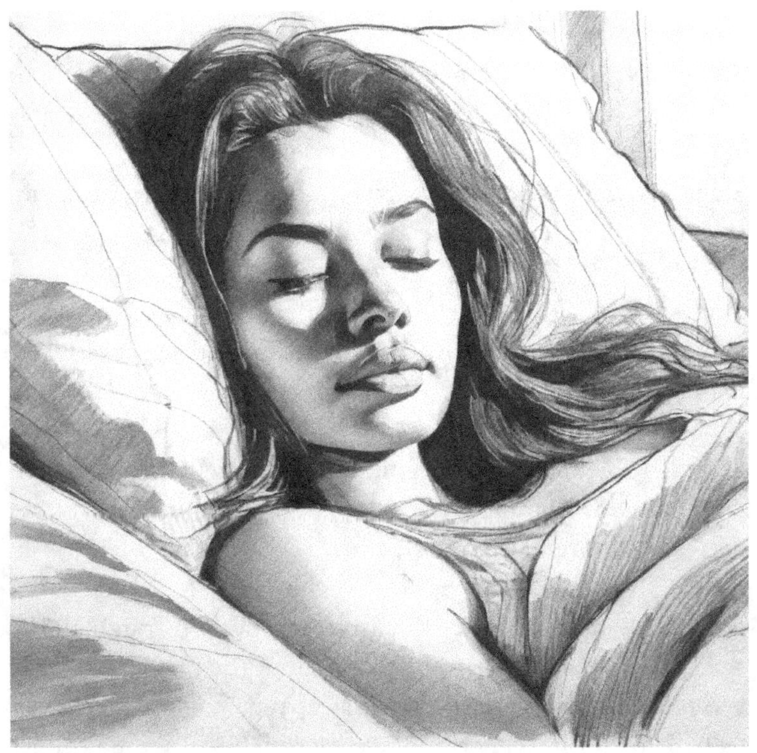

"Sleep is the silent orchestra orchestrating harmony within,

where dreams compose the symphony of understanding that the night whispers to our soul."

Sleep cycles and stages

Sleep follows a repeating cycle of non-REM (NREM) and REM (rapid eye movement) sleep stages that occur in a predictable order each night. There are 5 main stages:

Stage 1 NREM: The transition to sleep when heart rate and breathing slow slightly but brain activity is still high.

Stage 2 NREM: We become partially unconscious as brainwaves shift to larger, slower waves. Eye movement stops.

Stages 3 & 4 NREM (Delta Sleep): Brain activity slows even more and body temperature decreases. This is the deepest, most restorative sleep stage.

Stage 1 REM: Named for rapid eye movements, this is when vivid dreams commonly occur. Breathing and heart rate increase with reduced muscle tone.

It typically takes around 90 minutes to cycle through all the stages in a repeating pattern throughout the night. The early cycles focus more on NREM deep sleep repair, while later cycles feature longer REM periods. Most deep/NREM sleep occurs in the first half of the night, giving way to more REM in the later hours. Understanding these cycles helps optimize sleep conditions.

Factors that affect your sleep patterns

Here are some key factors that can affect individual sleep patterns:

- Age - Sleep cycles/needs change with development and aging. Teens/young adults need more, while older adults typically sleep less.

- Lifestyle - Exercise, diet, bedtimes, naps and daily routines all shape our internal clocks and sleep-wake cycles.

- Work schedule - Shift work, long hours, and inconsistent times disrupt circadian rhythms and sleep-wake regularity.

- Travel - Crossing time zones through travel impacts the body clock and makes it harder to fall/stay asleep when it thinks it's daytime.

- Illness/pain - Conditions like allergies, acid reflux, arthritis and restless legs can disturb sleep quality and continuity.

- Stress levels - Worry, grief, and mental health issues like anxiety and depression prevent relaxation and induce fragmented sleep.

- Sleep environment - Light, noise, temperature, mattress comfort and partner influences all affect sleep initiation and maintenance.

- Substance use - Coffee, alcohol and certain medications near bedtime have stimulating effects that deter deep slumber.

- Pregnancy - Hormonal changes, discomforts and the growing fetus affect sleep for expectant mothers.

Tracking lifestyle patterns alongside symptoms can uncover personal triggers affecting one's unique sleep-wake regulation. Subtle adjustments have profound effects when addressing root causes of poor quality sleep.

Indicators of sleep quality and quantity issues

Here are some common indicators that the quality or quantity of one's sleep may be compromised:

- Difficulty falling asleep or staying asleep through the night. This suggests struggles with sleep initiation or maintenance.

- Waking up earlier than desired and unable to fall back asleep. Could signal poor sleep efficiency.

- Oversleeping needs and still feeling unrefreshed upon waking. May point to an underlying sleep disorder.

- Daytime sleepiness like nodding off during sedentary activities or while driving. Sign of sleep debt build up.

- Mood changes such as irritability, impatience, anxiety and depression during the day. Inadequate sleep impacts mental well-being.

- Memory and concentration issues at work/school. Cognitive abilities hampered without sufficient deep sleep stages.

- Lack of energy and motivation to be active. Symptom of low energy levels from fragmented sleep patterns.

- Reliance on substances like coffee or occasional naps to power through the day. Compensating for poor overnight rest.

- Snoring, pauses in breathing or leg movements during sleep. Could be sleeping disorders needing treatment.

- Relationships/safety may be affected if sleepy during important functions. Risk of accidents increase with untreated sleep issues.

Paying attention to these potential red flags can uncover sleep problems early before serious impacts on health and wellness develop.

Assessing your individual sleep needs

Here are some effective ways to assess your individual sleep needs:

- Track how long and how well you've slept over a period of time via a sleep diary or wearable tracker. Note how refreshed you feel each morning.

- Look for optimum levels of deep NREM and REM sleep stages based on your age. Younger adults aged 18-25 typically need 7-9 hours per night.

- Note how long you feel fully functional during the day without a dip in energy levels or focus. This helps determine if you're getting enough duration and quality sleep.

- Try getting 30 extra minutes of sleep one night compared to your regular schedule. Compare mornings - do you feel significantly more refreshed with the longer duration?

- Consider napping needs. Only feeling a need to nap a few days per week suggests your overnight sleep is sufficiently restorative. Daily napping may signal sleep debt.

- Ask your doctor or sleep specialist to monitor factors like oxygen levels if you suspect an undiagnosed condition like sleep apnea. Testing sheds light on treatment options.

- Note effects on your mood and relationships. Quality sleep maintains balance and well-being which impacts all areas of life.

Regular evaluation customizes your wellness routine to fully meet your unique sleep needs at different life stages for optimal restorative benefits night after night.

Weekly Sleeping Tracker

Sleep Journal

Week of [Insert Start Date] to [Insert End Date]

Day 1: [Date]

- Bedtime: [Insert time]
    - Wake-up time: [Insert time]
    - Total Sleep Duration: [Calculate total hours]

Quality of Sleep:
    - [ ] Restful
    - [ ] Interrupted
    - [ ] Restless

Sleep Environment:
    - [ ] Quiet
    - [ ] Dark
    - [ ] Comfortable Temperature

Sleep Notes:
    [Insert any dreams, disturbances, or notable observations]

Day 2: [Date]

[Repeat the same format as Day 1 for the remaining days of the week.]

Weekly Summary:

Total Hours of Sleep:
   - Average: [Calculate average hours]
   - Highest Night: [Insert day and time]
   - Lowest Night: [Insert day and time]

Quality of Sleep:
   - [ ] Excellent
   - [ ] Good
   - [ ] Fair
   - [ ] Poor

Sleep Patterns:
   - [ ] Consistent bedtime
   - [ ] Consistent wake-up time
   - [ ] Irregular sleep schedule

Factors Affecting Sleep:
   - [ ] Stress
   - [ ] Caffeine intake
   - [ ] Exercise

Overall Feeling:
   - [ ] Energized
   - [ ] Tired
   - [ ] Neutral

Reflections:

[Optional section for thoughts on improvements, patterns, or changes to make for better sleep.]

Feel free to customize this template according to your preferences and add any additional details you find relevant.

Establishing a Bedtime Routine

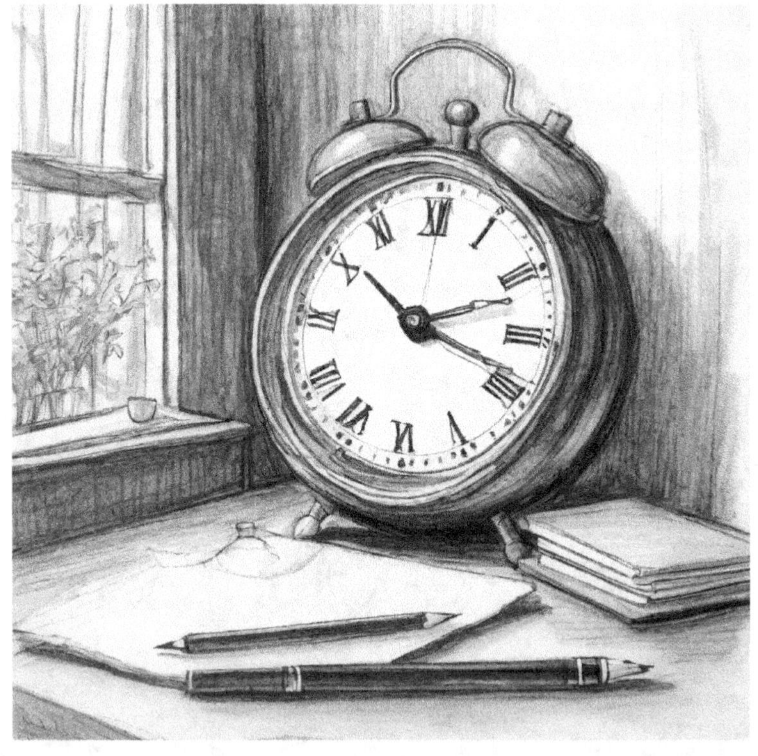

"Embrace the tranquility of night as you weave the threads of

routine, for in the simplicity of a bedtime ritual, you craft the masterpiece of restful dreams and rejuvenation."

Ways to wind down before bed

- Take a warm bath - The rise in body temperature from a bath triggers our internal thermostat to cool us off for sleep. Add Epsom salts or essential oils for extra relaxation.

- Gentle yoga or light stretches - Moving our bodies calmly before bed can work out kinks and lower stress levels. Focus on deep breathing during downward dog or child's pose.

- Read a book - Unplugging from screens in the hour before sleep allows our brain to shift focus using basic concentration and visual processing, unlike devices.

- Journal thoughts or plan tomorrow - Jotting down tasks and getting daily stresses "out of my head" has helped me fall asleep faster by clearing mental clutter.

- Sip chamomile or relaxation tea - Herbal teas like chamomile or sleepy time varieties contain compounds that can soothe nerves and promote drowsiness when the tea cools off.

- Listen to calming music - Try playlisting nature sounds, frequency tones or instrumental soothing genres on low volume through headphones or a speaker to relax both body and mind.

- Gentle massage - Rubbing essential oils like lavender or

gentle touches to tense areas releases feel-good hormones like serotonin that lull the nervous system.

Finding a wind-down routine you enjoy makes a difficult part of the day easier and improves your quality of rest ahead. Consistency is key for establishing good sleep habits.

Creating a calm, restful sleep environment

- Use blackout curtains or an eye mask to block any light from electronics or outdoor sources when sleeping. Melatonin production depends on darkness.

- Keep your bedroom cool. Most sleep experts recommend between 60-67°F for optimal temperature control as warmer can cause restlessness.

- Invest in a comfortable mattress and pillows suited to your body. Poor support alignment disrupts circulation and makes muscle relaxation difficult.

- Opt for light, breathable fabrics like cotton for bedding. Heavier materials can overheat the body. Avoid scented detergents with artificial fragrances that act as stimulants too close to the head.

- Clear clutter and dirty dishes from your bedroom so it feels clean, orderly and peaceful. Chaotic spaces add mental stimulation versus relaxation.

- Play white noise or nature sound playlists quietly in the background if outside interruptions bother you. Steady ambient sounds mask occasional noise disturbances.

- Use your bedroom only for sleep and sex to mentally associate it with rest. Ban electronics, late-night meals and stressful activities from disturbing that positive association.

- Consider blackout curtains, a box fan, humidifier or diffuser with calming essential oils to craft your perfect sleep microclimate. Adjust gadgets to the silent setting.

Paying attention to these sleep environment factors sets the stage for catching quality zzz's each and every night.

Developing a consistent sleep-wake schedule

Developing a consistent sleep-wake schedule is key for regulating your body's natural circadian rhythm and promoting quality sleep. Here are some tips for establishing routine:

- Pick set times to go to bed and wake up daily, even on weekends. Sticking to a 7-day schedule conditions your brain and hormones.

- Avoid daytime napping if possible, as short daytime sleep can disrupt nighttime sleep drive. If needed, limit naps to 30 minutes.

- Expose yourself to natural outdoor light throughout the day, especially in the morning. This helps set your body clock based on light and darkness cues.

- Cut off electronics one to two hours before bed since blue light suppresses melatonin production. Switch to low-stimulation activities instead.

- Establish a calming pre-bed routine like journaling, reading or a bath to inform your brain it's time to wind down mentally and physically.

- Make your bedroom only for sleep and sex so your body associates this environment with rest. Avoid stimulating activities in bed.

- Be patient, as it can take up to 3 weeks for your circadian rhythm to fully adjust. Sticking to the routine is key despite temptation to deviate or skip steps initially.

Consistency in your schedule and nighttime activities programs your body to expect sleep and achieve better quality rest over the long-term for overall health and wellness.

Reducing screen time and exposure to blue light

- Remove all screens (phone, TV, laptop etc.) at least 1-2 hours before bed to allow melatonin levels to rise naturally. The sooner the better.

- Install blue light filtering apps or adjust display settings on devices to reduce blue wavelength emissions in the evenings.

Alternatives include orange-tinted glasses.

- Limit recreational screen use to earlier in the day if possible to allot screen-free evening hours. Replace the habit with relaxing books, journaling or a hobby.

- Consider an electronic curfew for all non-essential devices like TVs and gaming consoles by a certain hour. Charge phones outside the bedroom overnight.

- If work requires evening screen use, take regular breaks to look into the distance and blink to re-orient eyes. Melatonin drops rapidly during breaks.

- Dimmer switches or table lamps are cozier lighting alternatives to overhead brights which impact circadian rhythms the least in the home at night.

- Read or do quiet activities before bed instead of exposure to stimulating device content and conversations that could flood the mind before trying to rest.

Implementing screen curfews and substitutes for mental wind-down promotes better sleep quality and longevity according to current research on impacts of blue wavelength light exposure.

Relaxing the Mind and Body for Better Sleep

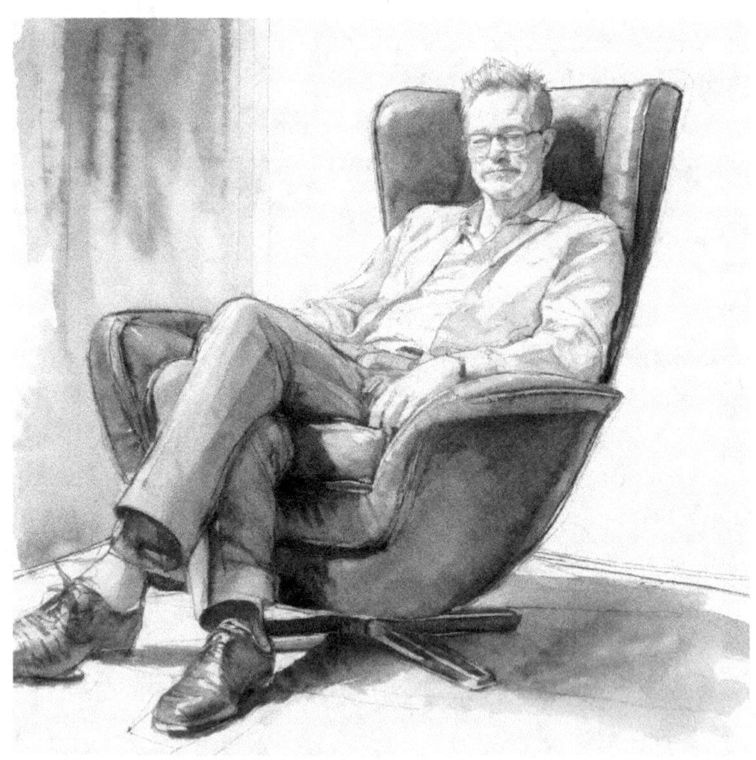

"In the quietude of serenity, let the mind unwind and the body soften; for in the gentle dance of relaxation, sleep finds its tranquil sanctuary, and dreams unfurl like petals in the night."

Stress management techniques

- Deep breathing: Taking slow, deep breaths engages the parasympathetic nervous system to lower stress levels. Apps like Insight Timer offer guided breathing sessions.

- Physical activity: As little as 10 minutes of light exercise per day like walking, yoga or stretching helps release endorphins and dissipate muscle tension from stress.

- Creative expression: Outlets like journaling, art, music, and cooking allow us to process emotions and anxieties through non-verbal means. The creative process induces calm.

- Social support: Talking with trusted friends or joining a support group puts stressors into perspective with a listening ear. Laughter and bonding also lower cortisol.

- Adequate sleep: Getting 7-9 hours nightly recharges our capacity to cope. Lack of sleep impairs emotional regulation and resilience under pressure.

- Mindfulness meditation: Apps like Calm guide meditation to help live in the present rather than dwelling on worries through non-judgmental awareness.

- Saying no: Letting go of perfectionism allows us to set boundaries without guilt when work or social obligations become too demanding on personal time and well-being.

- Healthy diet: Eating plenty of produce plus moderate complex carbs and proteins fuel both brain and body to thrive under stress instead of just surviving.

Finding what works best depends on individual personality and lifestyle, but consistency with stress relievers prevents burnout.

Gentle yoga and stretching before bed

Here are some gentle yoga poses and stretches one can do in the evenings to relax the body and mind before bed:

Child's Pose: From hands and knees, sit back on heels with forehead resting on the floor. Let hips sink and arms stretch out in front. Hold for 5 deep breaths to release lower back tension.

Reclined Bound Angle Pose: Lying on your back, bring the soles of feet together with knees falling outward like a "M". Clasp hands around knees and breathe into tight hips and hamstrings.

Shoulder Circles: Standing tall, drawing slow circles forward and back with shoulders to loosen tight neck and upper back muscles from time spent hunched over screens.

Cat-Cow: On hands and knees, inhale to drop belly and look up for cow pose, then exhale rounding through upper back into cat pose for gentle spinal flexion.

Pigeon Pose: Bringing one knee forward then sliding the same side arm back, pressing the bent front leg open to feel a stretch through outer hips and glutes.

Legs Up the Wall: Ending in total relaxation by propping hips against a wall with legs extended up for an inversion soothing the whole body.

Breathing consciously into any tight areas throughout allows tension to dissipate as we prepare physically and mentally for stillness and restoration overnight. Gentle yet effective!

Mindfulness and meditation practices

Body Scan Meditation - Starting from the toes and slowly sweeping attention up through muscle groups, this allows detection of physical tension holding stress.

Breath Focus - Simple awareness of the natural breathing cycle, observing the rise and fall without controlling it. When mind wanders, gently return focus.

Gratitude Practice - Jotting down things one feels grateful for in a journal every evening cultivates an appreciative mindset.

Loving Kindness Meditation - Silently repeating phrases like "May I be happy, healthy, and at peace" to develop compassion for oneself and others.

Walking Meditation - Mindfully noting sensations as feet contact the ground, observing feelings and thoughts from a distanced perspective.

Sound Meditation - Focusing intently on ambient noises such as traffic, nature or chimes to practice presence without conceptual thinking.

Listening to Guided Meditations - Apps and online recordings offer guided introductions to mindfulness and support building a regular practice.

Consistency is key, even starting with just 5-10 minutes daily of silent presence has lasting effects on stress, focus, relationships and overall well-being. Perspective is a powerful tool for navigating life's ebbs and flows.

Nutrition and Lifestyle Strategies for Quality Sleep

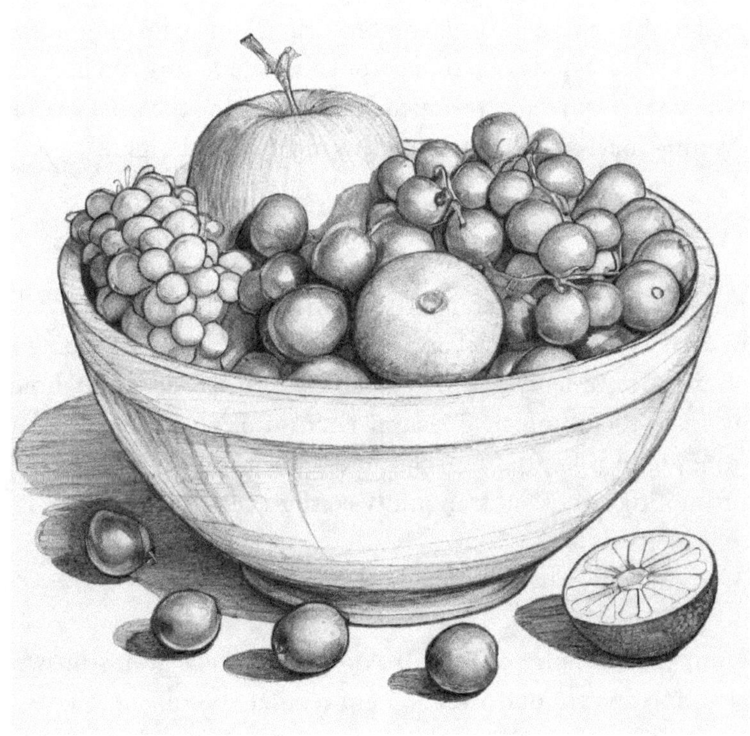

"Nourish the night with mindful choices, where the symphony of sleep is composed by the harmonious notes of nutrition and lifestyle; for in the rhythm of well-being, dreams find their richest melodies."

The role of diet in sleep

1. Tryptophan: The Precursor to Serenity

At the heart of the diet-sleep connection lies tryptophan, an amino acid that serves as a precursor to serotonin and melatonin—two neurotransmitters crucial for regulating sleep-wake cycles. Foods rich in tryptophan include turkey, chicken, nuts, seeds, and dairy products. Incorporating these into your evening meals may contribute to a more restful night.

2. The Magnesium Marvel

Magnesium, often referred to as nature's relaxant, plays a pivotal role in muscle and nerve function. It's found in abundance in leafy green vegetables, nuts, seeds, and whole grains. Including magnesium-rich foods in your diet can potentially relax the muscles and calm the nervous system, promoting a sense of tranquility conducive to sleep.

3. Complex Carbohydrates: Fuel for the Night

Opting for complex carbohydrates, such as whole grains, brown rice, and sweet potatoes, can help regulate blood sugar levels throughout the night. These slow-releasing carbohydrates provide a sustained energy source, preventing blood sugar spikes and crashes that may disrupt sleep.

4. The Caffeine Conundrum

While a cup of coffee might be your morning ally, its stimulating effects can linger for hours. It's wise to limit caffeine intake in the afternoon and evening to avoid interference with your body's natural wind-down process. Swap that late-night espresso for a soothing herbal tea to promote a more peaceful transition to sleep.

5. Timing Matters: The Art of Meal Timing

The timing of meals can influence sleep quality. Consuming heavy or spicy meals too close to bedtime may lead to discomfort and indigestion. Aim for a balanced dinner at least a few hours before bedtime, allowing your body ample time to digest before you hit the hay.

Hydration and avoiding late-night drinks

1. The Water-Weave: Hydration and Sleep Harmony

Proper hydration is not only essential for overall health but is intricately tied to our sleep patterns. Dehydration can lead to discomfort, prompting sleep interruptions as the body strives to signal its need for fluids. Establishing a consistent water intake throughout the day helps maintain optimal hydration levels, setting the stage for a more comfortable night's rest.

2. Timing Matters: The Hydration Equation

While drinking enough water during the day is vital, being mindful of your intake closer to bedtime can make a significant difference. Consuming large quantities of fluids right before bed may lead to disruptive midnight trips to the bathroom, disrupting the continuity of your sleep. Aim to taper off your water consumption in the evening, finding a balance that keeps you hydrated without causing nocturnal disturbances.

3. Caffeine and Nighttime Nuisance

Late-night drinks often come with hidden sleep disruptors, and caffeine is a prime culprit. Tea, coffee, and certain sodas contain caffeine, a stimulant that can linger in the system for hours. Opting for caffeine-free herbal teas or warm water with a hint of lemon in the evening can be a soothing alternative, providing hydration without the risk of unwanted wakefulness.

4. Alcohol's Deceptive Drowsiness

While alcohol may initially induce drowsiness, its impact on sleep cycles is more complex. It can interfere with the deeper stages of sleep, leading to fragmented and less restorative rest. Limiting alcohol consumption, especially in the hours leading up to bedtime, can contribute to a more peaceful and rejuvenating night.

5. The Ritual of Relaxation: Herbal Infusions and Warm Water

As an alternative to stimulants, consider incorporating calming herbal infusions into your evening routine. Chamomile, valerian root, and peppermint teas are known for their relaxation-inducing properties. Sipping on warm water can also have a calming effect, promoting a sense of tranquility before you tuck yourself in.

Exercise and activity levels

We all know that exercise is important for our physical and mental health, but did you know the timing and type of workouts you do can significantly influence the quality of your sleep as well? As a passionate yoga teacher and jogger, I'm well aware of how activity rhythms sync up with my body's natural circadian processes. Here are some insights into maximizing exercise's sleep-boosting potential based on my own active lifestyle experiments over the years.

Cardiovascular exercise performed regularly during daylight hours is ideal for the greatest sleep benefits. The moderate increase in core temperature and elevated heart rate fires up stress hormone production which needs to fully dissipate before bed. Allowing 2-3 hours after your workout for a natural cooldown is key so you don't enter an overtired state that can disrupt the onset of sleepiness cues later in the evening.

Personally, I find outdoor jogging in early to midafternoon works perfectly as it raises my energy levels to stay focused and productive without lingering effects when nightfall arrives. However, morning is better than late at night for those less active folks to guarantee exercise fatigue has sufficiently resolved before hitting the sack.

While gentle yoga or stretching can relax tight muscles right before sleeping, more intense sessions too close to bed may induce aches and pains as the body processes lactic acid buildup. For me, an evening vinyasa flow is pleasantly stimulating followed by restorative poses to let tension seep away gradually. Saving higher energy workouts earlier optimizes this natural winding down process supported by exercise.

Establishing consistent activity patterns also regulates your circadian clocks to anticipate sleepiness and alertness triggers predictably. Sticking to a regular routine benefits my sleep quality tremendously versus days blowing it all off until nightfall with disruptive consequences. Finding what timing and types suit your lifestyle best takes trial and error but pays dividends in more refreshing rest.

With some adjustments, we can leverage daytime workouts as a natural inducer of slumber's sweet release every night. It's about listening to your body's rhythms and honoring recovery throughout this cycle for peak physical and mental functioning overall.

Caffeine, nicotine and other substances

Here is a 500-word draft article on how caffeine, nicotine and other substances impact sleep:

Caffeine, Smokes and Your Sleep: The Effects of Stimulants

As a writer and fitness coach, optimal sleep is key to keeping up with my busy lifestyle while staying energized and focused throughout long workdays. However, indulging certain vices was jeopardizing my quality of rest, sparking some in-depth research on stimulants' sleep-stealing abilities. By sharing what I learned, I hope to help others improve their zzz's too through properly timed enjoyment.

Let's start with caffeine, my former arch nemesis after years of coffee dependency. Lasting 6-8 hours in your system, even just one cup four hours before bed significantly inhibits melatonin release and leaves half the caffeine floating around later at night. Switching to half-caff by 3 p.m. and tea/decaf by evening did the trick for me when breaking the habit was too harsh. Knowing its duration means planning intake wisely well in advance of lights out.

Similarly, those evening nicotine cravings from smoking pack quite a stimulating wallop. Even third-hand smoke stuck to clothes retains enough drugs disrupting dreams through clothing fibers brought indoors. Try vaping once work ends and waiting several hours before snoozing while wearing a fresh outfit to bed. Gradually reducing daily use may even enhance your sleep depth long term according to studies.

Stress releases cortisol tricking you to stay up late worrying or doom scrolling versus taking restorative downtime earlier on. Mellowing out mindfulness practices and breathing exercises work better for me than TV and screens heating up my nervous system too close to bedtime afterwards.

Using stimulants sensibly takes practice to dial in properly for your lifestyle and needs. I've found caffeine, smokes and stress not avoided altogether but enjoyed earlier serves my energy levels and sleep much better versus late indulgence as the adage goes - everything in moderation!

Common Sleep Disorders

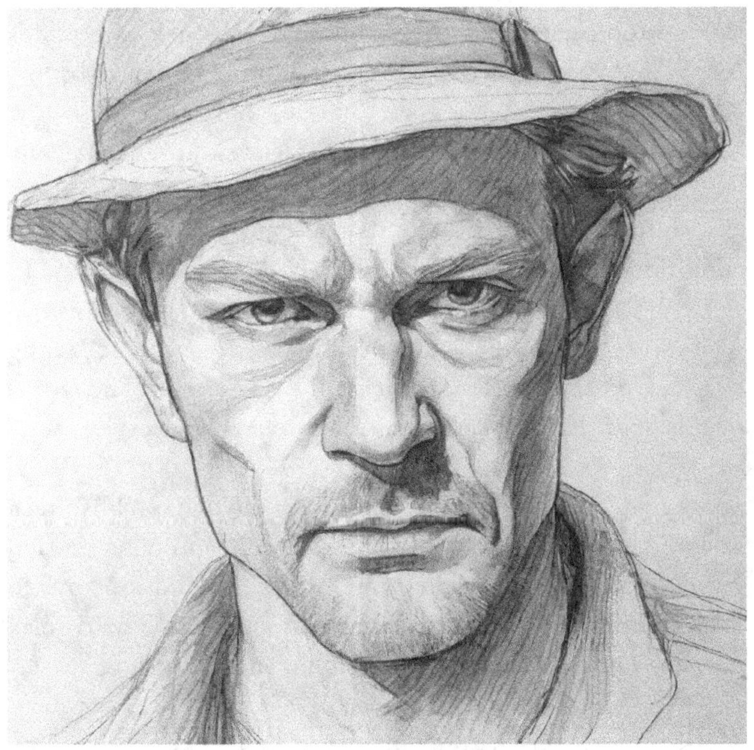

"In the realm of the night, a disorderly dance of restlessness

unfolds, where dreams and wakefulness blur, revealing the intricate tapestry of a sleep disrupted but not defeated."

Insomnia

As someone who has suffered occasional bouts of insomnia myself, I've gained a fair understanding of what causes this elusive sleep disorder and what helps alleviate symptoms:

Insomnia refers to difficulty falling asleep, staying asleep, or waking too early and not being able to fall back asleep. It's considered chronic if symptoms last more than 3 months.

Stress, anxiety, depression, and hyperactive thinking are common triggers that keep the mind racing even in bed. Additionally, shifts in work schedules, screens before bed, and medical conditions can disrupt normal sleep patterns.

At its worst, insomnia is exasperating and leaves one feeling fatigued yet unable to nap during the day either. The worry over lack of sleep exacerbates itself into a vicious cycle.

Some remedies I've found success with include establishing a relaxing bedtime routine, limiting caffeine and naps, getting natural light in the mornings, practicing meditation apps to declutter thoughts, light exercise earlier in the day to relax muscles, and avoiding screens/stimuli before winding down.

Melatonin or herbal supplements may help reset circadian clocks short-term too under doctor guidance. Most importantly, not stressing about sleep helps get past overthinking it as psychological factors play a big role.

With time and consistency in healthy habits, even chronic insomnia can usually substantially improve quality of life. The solutions are not one size fits all though, so it takes self awareness to find what methods work best.

Sleep apnea

Sleep apnea is a potentially serious sleep disorder where breathing repeatedly stops and starts throughout the night due to collapsed airways. There are two main types - obstructive, caused by throat muscle relaxation, and central, due to brain malfunction.

Watching my late father struggle with loud snoring and erratic breathing spells that would jolt him awake in a panic was distressing. His exhaustion was also always evident yet naps brought no relief. Thankfully his doctor took concerns seriously to diagnose obstructive sleep apnea through an overnight sleep study.

Dad was prescribed a CPAP machine to provide steady air pressure and keep his throat propped open as he slept. This device greatly improved his quality of rest once he adjusted to the unfamiliar sensation. Foggy morning headaches vanished along with daytime drowsiness over time with consistent nightly use.

Sleep apnea robs the body of oxygen and disrupts sleep cycles, which wears down the organs and cardiovascular system if left untreated. Early screening is important since it often goes undiagnosed. While an inconvenience to use equipment, the health risks like diabetes, stroke and heart attack it can provoke are no joke. I'm grateful modern solutions exist to support restorative slumber for folks suffering from this common yet serious sleep disruption. Raising awareness is key so no one else has to endure its debilitating effects.

Restless legs syndrome

Restless Legs Syndrome (RLS) involves unpleasant, tingling or prickly sensations deep in the legs and an irresistible urge to move them - often worse at night - interfering with sleep quality. Around 1 in 20 experience this neurological disorder to varying degrees.

The cause is not fully understood but seems linked to imbalances of dopamine, a chemical messenger in the brain regulating movement and deep rest. Some key symptoms include worsening discomfort when sitting still like lectures or movies, fleeting relief with walking breaks, and sensations moving up the body over time.

While not typically debilitating for everyone, severe sufferers understandably dread bedtime grappling with distractions from disturbing limb vibrations. Treatments involve iron and dopamine supplements, massage and stretching during flare-ups plus hot baths for soothing effects.

I've seen the joy when simple fixes significantly calm patient's legs enough for relieving rest. However, in stubborn chronic cases resistant to conservative methods, specialists may trial prescription therapies such as low-dose meds, injections or nerve stimulators as a last resort.

Overall raising awareness about this misunderstood yet common condition's frustrating physical and emotional impacts is important. Appropriate screening and targeted non-drug remedies enhance life quality for anyone dealing with restless nights due to their tormenting tinglers.

Narcolepsy

Narcolepsy involves an overpowering need to sleep during the daytime due to faulty brain mechanisms regulating wakefulness. It stems from a lack of a neurotransmitter called hypocretin that sends alertness signals. Symptoms often begin in the late teens/early 20s and include:

- Daytime drowsiness making it difficult to stay focused or functional without frequent naps. The constant fatigue can take a huge mental/emotional toll.

- Sleep attacks where sudden irresistible sleepiness strikes at inopportune moments like conversations or driving, causing "sleep drunkenness" spells.

- Hallucinations between sleeping and waking that are vivid yet frightening.

- Cataplexy - complete or partial muscle weakness/paralysis triggered by strong emotions like laughter that can cause collapse without injury.

Diagnosis involves overnight sleep studies combined with spinal fluid tests. While there is no cure, prescription drugs can help reduce symptoms along with proper sleep hygiene, stress management, exercise, light exposure and avoiding trigger situations.

Living with narcolepsy takes immense courage as one learns delicate balance between rest and responsibilities. Treatment and support groups uplift patients dealing with unique set of challenges to daily life that many do not comprehend. Spreading awareness of this neurological disorder is crucial.

Putting It All Together

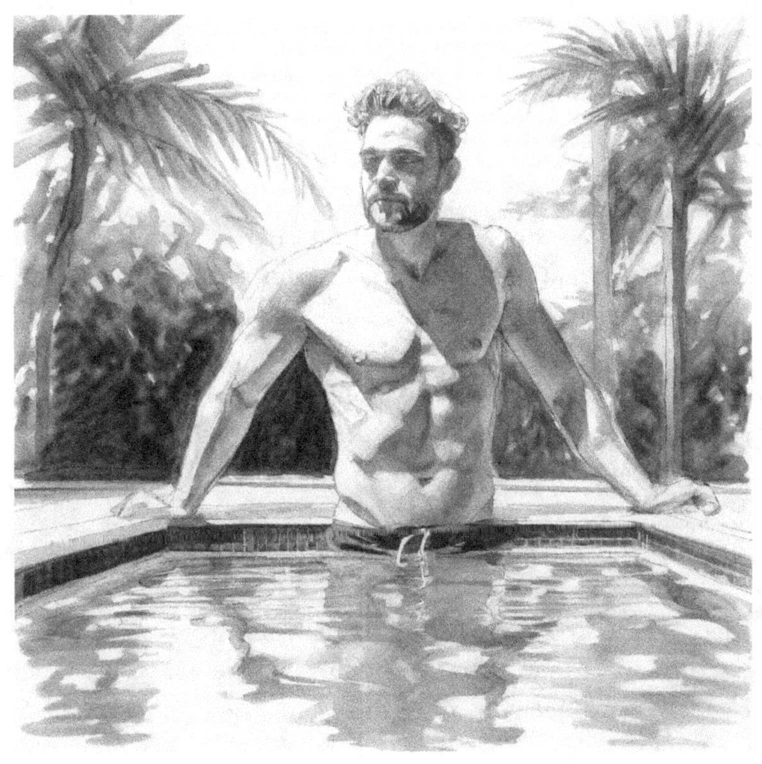

Customizing a self-care routine for better sleep

1. Reflecting on Rest: Understanding Your Sleep Needs

Before delving into the world of self-care, take a moment to reflect on your sleep patterns and needs. Consider the factors that may be contributing to restlessness or sleep disruptions. Are there specific stressors, environmental factors, or lifestyle habits that could be affecting your sleep? Understanding these aspects lays the foundation for a targeted and effective self-care routine.

2. Crafting a Calming Bedtime Ritual

Bedtime rituals signal to your body that it's time to wind down and prepare for sleep. Tailor your routine to activities that calm and relax you. This could include activities such as reading a book, practicing gentle stretches, or engaging in a few minutes of mindfulness meditation. Experiment with different elements until you find a combination that resonates with you and cultivates a sense of tranquility.

3. The Power of Pampering: Skincare and Relaxation

Incorporating skincare into your evening routine not only nurtures your skin but also becomes a luxurious act of self-care. Experiment with soothing scents, such as lavender or chamomile-infused products, to create a sensory experience that promotes relaxation. Taking the time for a warm bath or shower can further enhance the pampering effect, preparing both body and mind for restful sleep.

4. Tech Detox: Unplugging for Uninterrupted Sleep

The glow of screens can disrupt the body's natural circadian rhythm. Consider implementing a tech detox at least an hour before bedtime. This means putting away smartphones, tablets, and computers to allow your brain to transition into a state of relaxation. Instead, opt for calming activities that don't involve screens, such as listening to soothing music or practicing gentle yoga.

5. Nourishing Nighttime: Mindful Eating for Better Sleep

The foods we consume can impact our sleep quality. Experiment with incorporating sleep-friendly snacks into your evening routine. Foods rich in tryptophan, magnesium, and complex carbohydrates, such as a small serving of yogurt with nuts or a banana, can contribute to a more restful night. Be mindful of portion sizes and avoid heavy meals close to bedtime.

6. Creating a Comfortable Sleep Sanctuary

Evaluate your sleep environment to ensure it promotes relaxation. Consider factors such as room temperature, lighting, and the comfort of your mattress and pillows. Customizing your sleep space to align with your preferences can enhance the overall effectiveness of your self-care routine.

Overcoming obstacles and maintaining changes

1. Identifying the Culprits: Unmasking Sleep Obstacles

Before implementing changes, it's crucial to identify the specific obstacles standing in the way of restful sleep. Common culprits include stress, irregular sleep schedules, excessive screen time, and unhealthy lifestyle habits. Take stock of your daily routine and pinpoint the factors that may be sabotaging your sleep quality.

2. Stress Management: Unwinding the Mind for Sleep

Stress is a formidable adversary to restful sleep. Integrate stress-management techniques into your daily routine, such as mindfulness meditation, deep breathing exercises, or gentle yoga. Cultivating a practice that helps you unwind and let go of the day's tensions can significantly contribute to a more tranquil bedtime.

3. Establishing Consistent Sleep Patterns: A Rhythm of Rest

The body thrives on routine, and establishing consistent sleep patterns reinforces its natural circadian rhythm. Aim for a regular bedtime and wake-up time, even on weekends. This consistency helps regulate your internal clock, making it easier to fall asleep and wake up naturally.

4. Screen-Time Curfew: Dimming the Disruptions

The glow of screens, be it from smartphones, tablets, or computers, can interfere with the production of melatonin, a hormone essential for sleep. Implement a screen-time curfew at least an hour before bedtime. Engage in calming activities instead, such as reading a physical book or practicing gentle stretches.

5. Creating a Comfortable Sleep Environment: The Sanctuary of Sleep

Evaluate your sleep environment to ensure it promotes relaxation. Keep the room dark, quiet, and cool. Invest in a comfortable mattress and pillows. Creating a sleep sanctuary enhances the likelihood of restful nights and reinforces positive changes over the long term.

6. Healthy Lifestyle Choices: Fueling Sleep with Nutrition

Nutrition plays a crucial role in sleep quality. Be mindful of caffeine and heavy meals close to bedtime. Opt for sleep-friendly snacks, such as a small serving of yogurt or a handful of nuts, to support a more restful night. Maintaining a balanced diet contributes not only to overall health but also to sustained improvements in sleep.

7. Tracking Progress: The Power of Sleep Journals

Keeping a sleep journal allows you to track progress, identify patterns, and make informed adjustments to your routine. Note bedtime, wake-up time, sleep quality, and any notable factors affecting your sleep. This valuable tool helps you stay accountable and fine-tune your approach over time.

8. Seeking Professional Guidance: When Obstacles Persist

If obstacles persist despite your efforts, consider seeking professional guidance. A healthcare provider or sleep specialist can offer tailored advice, conduct assessments, and explore potential underlying issues that may be hindering your sleep.

Achieving holistic wellness through quality sleep

1. The Foundations of Holistic Wellness: Sleep as a Cornerstone

Holistic wellness encompasses more than just physical health—it embraces the interconnectedness of mind, body, and spirit. Quality sleep serves as a cornerstone in this intricate balance, influencing everything from cognitive function and emotional resilience to immune system strength and overall vitality.

2. Cognitive Clarity: Sharpening the Mind Through Restful Sleep

A well-rested mind is a clear and focused mind. Quality sleep enhances cognitive functions such as memory consolidation, problem-solving, and creativity. Prioritizing adequate sleep contributes to improved mental clarity, allowing you to navigate daily challenges with a heightened sense of awareness and resilience.

3. Emotional Resilience: Nurturing Mental Well-being

The impact of sleep on emotional well-being is profound. Sleep deprivation can heighten stress levels and negatively affect mood regulation. On the contrary, quality sleep provides the emotional resilience needed to navigate life's ups and downs with a greater sense of balance and composure.

4. Physical Restoration: Strengthening the Body from Within

During sleep, the body undergoes essential processes of repair and regeneration. Hormones are released, muscles are repaired, and the immune system is strengthened. Prioritizing quality sleep sets the stage for physical well-being, contributing to increased energy levels, faster recovery from exercise, and a fortified immune system.

5. Hormonal Harmony: Balancing Vital Functions

Sleep plays a pivotal role in hormonal balance, influencing crucial functions such as appetite regulation, metabolism, and stress response. Disruptions in sleep patterns can lead to hormonal imbalances, potentially contributing to weight gain, increased stress, and other health issues. Consistent, quality sleep fosters hormonal harmony, promoting overall wellness.

6. Establishing Healthy Sleep Hygiene: A Ritual of Self-Care

Creating a routine that supports quality sleep is an act of self-care that reverberates throughout your entire well-being. Establishing a regular sleep schedule, cultivating a calming bedtime routine, and optimizing your sleep environment are essential components of healthy sleep hygiene.

7. Mind-Body Connection: Sleep as a Spiritual Practice

In the pursuit of holistic wellness, recognizing the mind-body connection is paramount. Quality sleep nurtures not only the physical and mental aspects but also serves as a form of spiritual replenishment. Embracing sleep as a sacred practice aligns the spiritual dimension, fostering a sense of inner peace and connectedness.

8. The Long-Term Impact: Sustaining Holistic Wellness Through Sleep

Achieving holistic wellness is not a destination but an ongoing journey. Prioritizing quality sleep isn't just a short-term fix; it's a commitment to sustained well-being. As sleep becomes an integral part of your lifestyle, its transformative effects permeate every facet of your life, contributing to a harmonious and balanced existence.

Conclusion

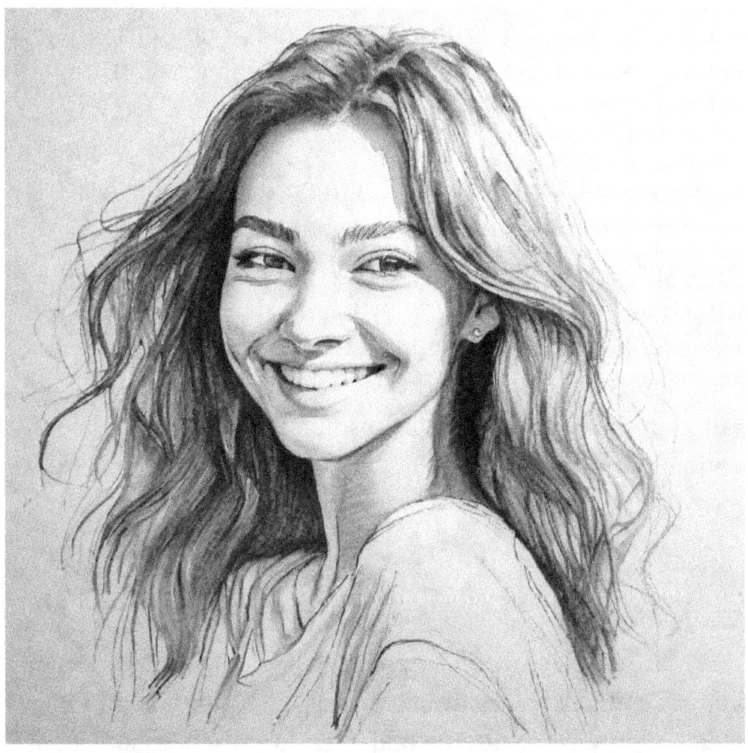

As avid athletes, performers, entrepreneurs, and all-around hustlers, many of us take pride in our ability to maximize every minute of the day. However, our fast-paced lifestyles often come at the detriment of our most important natural function - sleep. As the old proverb goes, "The busy man is not half as busy as he thinks he is. He has lots of time to think."

While thinking has its place during daylight hours, mental stimulation before bed prevents true relaxation and restoration overnight. As difficult as it may be, unwinding our overactive minds is essential for health, productivity and overall well-being in the long run. With awareness and commitment to small changes, we can overcome habits keeping us from slumber's sweet embrace night after night.

In this concluding section, I aim to synthesize effective strategies for sleeping your way to the top based on insights from modern science, ancient wisdom traditions, and strategies that keep this writer and entrepreneur well-rested through countless deadlines and adrenaline-fueled days. It takes vigilance and patience to replace obstacles with optimizing behaviors, but your mind and body will absolutely thank you as benefits compound over time.

Major Lifestyle Changes

While screens are a leading cause of disrupted sleep for obvious reasons, other lifestyle factors warrant examination and adjustment. Excessive intake of caffeine, alcohol, and heavy meals all interfere with the body's natural rhythms and signals for resting. As does inconsistent sleep schedules on weekends paired with early rise times expected on weekdays. It's no wonder we struggle drifting off or staying asleep!

For lasting transformation, I recommend thoughtfully analyzing your daily habits to identify potential problem areas sabotaging seven to nine hours of quality slumber nightly. This could mean setting a firm cutoff time for caffeinated beverages at 3pm instead of a last-minute 10pm coffee. Or committing to making dinner your largest meal so digestion wraps up well before lights out. And of course, honoring the same bed and wake windows consistently seven days a week.

It takes diligence to establish new routines that serve rather than hinder the needs of your inner circadian clock. Refer to checklists, calendar reminders or enlist an accountability buddy if adherence feels daunting at first. The gradual process is worth sleep rewards paying dividends for focus, health, joy and success. Rome wasn't built in a day, so focus on consistency over perfection as changes take hold.

Cutting Blue Light Before Bed

While certain screens stir slumber woes, the blue wavelength light they emit specifically suppresses our production of sleep-inducing melatonin hormone at critical pre-bedtime hours. Luckily, technology now offers solutions to combat this modern curse.

Some apps like f.lux or Iris for Apple automatically adjust devices to warmer colors reducing blue light exposure later in the day and evenings as the sun sets. On Android, Night Shift serves a similar purpose when enabled. Blue light blocking glasses specifically designed for computers and phones provide protection whether adjusting digital settings or not.

For screens off the bedside table, smart bulbs or lighting strips help shine softer amber tones around the home instead of sterile whites stimulating brainwaves as night falls. Candlelight creates calming dim atmospheres ideal for settling in without devices altogether.

The key is avoiding blue light sources as much as realistically possible in the hour or two before hitting the hay, allowing your pineal gland to produce its full supply of cozy melatonin without disruption. Noticing the difference this golden glow makes feels absolutely brilliant!

Pre-Sleep Calm & Relaxation

While certain screens stir slumber woes, the blue wavelength light they emit specifically suppresses our production of sleep-inducing melatonin hormone at critical pre-bedtime hours. Luckily, technology now offers solutions to combat this modern curse.

Some apps like f.lux or Iris for Apple automatically adjust devices to warmer colors reducing blue light exposure later in the day and evenings as the sun sets. On Android, Night Shift serves a similar purpose when enabled. Blue light blocking glasses specifically designed for computers and phones provide protection whether adjusting digital settings or not.

For screens off the bedside table, smart bulbs or lighting strips help shine softer amber tones around the home instead of sterile whites stimulating brainwaves as night falls. Candlelight creates calming dim atmospheres ideal for settling in without devices altogether.

The key is avoiding blue light sources as much as realistically possible in the hour or two before hitting the hay, allowing your pineal gland to produce its full supply of cozy melatonin without disruption. Noticing the difference this golden glow makes feels absolutely brilliant!

Pre-Sleep Calm & Relaxation

Setting aside screen time allows applying soothing activities to unwind our mental chatter. Some favorites of mine include practicing gratitude journaling, shadow work journaling to dump worries, taking a bath with epsom salts + essential oils, and listening to guided meditations or calming audiobooks. Deep breathing techniques, mindfulness meditation, and gentle yoga flows are wonderfully tranquilizing as well.

On nights when thoughts run wild, I've found progressive muscle relaxation scripts particularly helpful. Starting with tensing groups like fingers to toes then releasing one by one induces mental as well as physical loosening. Visualizing a rejuvenating slumber scene while concentrating on each body region loosens hold of anxious thinking. Amazing how something so simple can feel so restorative.

For me, nourishing myself with nourishing nourishment like chamomile tea, herbal nighttime supplements or calming foods enhances relaxation further. Tart cherry jam/dried fruit, tart cherry juice, eggs, turkey, fish, nuts/seeds provide tryptophan boosting serotonin and melatonin hormones naturally. Binaural beats or solfeggio frequency music helps shift brainwaves through headphones as needed too.

The goal is releasing tension completely both mentally and physically so there's nothing left for the mind to latch onto restlessly once under covers. This primes you to slip seamlessly into sleep's serenity. With patient practice, unwinding becomes second nature before the best part of day arrives.

Creating an Ideal Sleep Sanctuary

Now that lifestyle and mindset support restorative slumber, focus shifts to cultivating an ideal bedroom oasis. This starts with lightproofing curtains or an eye mask, white noise machine or fan, perhaps some cozy fabrics, nourishing scents like lavender, and ideally nature sounds or chill sleep meditations playing softly via Bluetooth speaker.

Blackout prevents wake-ups from natural light or neighbors, white noise drowns disruptive noises, luxurious linens and fluffy pillows form a refuge, and soothing aromas carry our consciousness tranquilly to the dreamworld. You absolutely wouldn't want distractions here!

I also enjoy using temperature regulating bedding and a cooling pillow to sync metabolism with the cooler evening hours ideal for sleep triggering thermoregulation. My mattress sees seasonal updates to suit changed bodies and sleeping positions too. Whatever enhances coziness and promotes quality rest receives consideration.

Setting this nurturing sleep sanctuary invites full relaxation so challenging thoughts melt away naturally. You start looking forward to bedtime not dreading it, eager to immerse in the precious healing it offers. Naturally with a place this inviting, slumber comes easily as a welcome guest each night.

Consistency Is Crucial

While implementing strategic lifestyle shifts optimizes conditions for better sleep, consistency in honoring your natural circadian rhythms proves most important. Establishing a set schedule, sticking to wind-down and bedtime routines, avoiding irregular sleep-wake patterns - these ensure hormonal and biological processes stay regulated as they were designed.

As busy individuals constantly bouncing between tasks, places and time zones, maintaining homeostasis in our routines requires determination. But powering through short-term disruptions and committing to best practices pays huge long-term dividends in sustainable restorative sleep and peak functioning. It has truly changed my energy levels, resilience and productivity tenfold.

Whether adjusting slowly on weekends or sticking rigidly to clockwork sleep-wake windows seven days a week while traveling, honoring your body's needs through consistency rewards greatly. Consistency is said to be the hobgoblin of little minds, but it seems to serve the overactive mind and hardworking body brilliantly in shutting down each evening on time. Such a worthwhile investment you can't put a price on!

While systemic obstacles like shift work, health issues or un-supportive sleep environments pose difficulty, small sacrifices do make a difference. Analyzing what impedes our best rest and gradually optimizing gives great control over the quality of unconscious hours. This improves every facet of living tremendously.

As ambitious people settling into bed earlier each night might feel counterintuitive or boring. But this extra dose of slumber supercharges our days, sharpens focus, lifts mood, fortifies health and regenerates our drive to accomplish even more. It enhances productivity far beyond late nights ever could. Plus, waking refreshed gives more enjoyment from each moment.

Though demanding lifestyles tempt disregarding nature's sleep patterns, maintaining homeostasis through discipline pays dividends. With awareness of triggers and implementing techniques at our own pace, nourishing slumber becomes second nature. Then we flow effortlessly through goals powered by perpetual renewal each morning - the true key to hustling sustainably and success on our own terms. Sweet dreams ahead to all!